BREAD MACHINE COOKBOOK

Hands-off Recipes for
perfect Homemade Bread

DAN RIDOLFI

Table of Contents

Introduction

Bread making machine, otherwise known as a bread maker, is a home-based appliance that transforms uncooked ingredients into bread. It is made up of a saucepan for bread (or "tin"), with one or more built-in paddles at the bottom, present in the center of a small special-purpose oven. This little oven is usually operated via a control panel via a simple in-built computer utilizing the input settings. Some bread machines have diverse cycles for various forms of dough — together with white bread, whole grain, European-style (occasionally called "French"), and dough-only (for pizza dough and formed loaves baked in a traditional oven). Many also have a timer to enable the bread machine to work without the operator's attendance, and some high-end models allow the user to program a customized period.

To bake bread, ingredients are measured in a specified order into the bread pan (usually first liquids, with solid ingredients layered on top), and then the pan is put in the bread maker. The order of ingredients is important because contact with water triggers the instant yeast used in bread makers, so the yeast and water have to be kept separate until the program starts.

It takes the machine several hours to make a bread loaf. The products are rested first and brought to an optimal temperature. Stir with a paddle, and the ingredients are then shaped into a flour. Use optimal temperature regulation, and the dough is then confirmed and then cooked.

When the bread has been baked, the bread maker removes the pan. Then leaving a slight indentation from the rod to which the paddle is connected. The finished loaf's shape is often regarded as unique. Many initial bread machines manufacture a vertically slanted towards, square, or cylindrical loaf that is significantly dissimilar from commercial bread; however, more recent units typically have a more conventional horizontal pan. Some bread machines use two paddles to form two lb. loaf in regular rectangle shape.

Bread machine recipes are often much smaller than regular bread recipes. Sometimes standardized based on the machine's pan capacity, most popular in the US market is 1.5 lb./700 g units. Most recipes are written for that capacity; however, two lb./900 g units are not uncommon. There are prepared bread mixes, specially made for bread makers, containing pre-measured ingredients and flour and yeast, flavorings, and sometimes dough conditioners.

Bread makers are also fitted with a timer for testing when bread-making starts. For example, this allows them to be loaded at night but only begin baking in the morning to produce a freshly baked bread for breakfast. They may also be set only for making dough, for example, for making pizza. Apart from bread, some can also be set to make other things like jam, pasta dough, and Japanese rice cake. Some of the new developments in the facility of the machine includes automatically adding nut. It also contains fruit from a tray during the kneading process. Bread makers typically take between three and four hours to bake a loaf. However, recent "quick bake" modes have become standard additions, many of which can produce a loaf in less than an hour.

The History of Bread

We forget to sometimes conceptualize the beginning of many of the items we have labelled 'regular' within our daily lives. The same goes for bread, which is said to have originated in 8,000 BC from the areas surrounding Egypt.

However, bread in the form that we can recognize today may have shared links with Chapatis as it is known in India, and perhaps the classic

Tortilla that is well-known in Mexico.

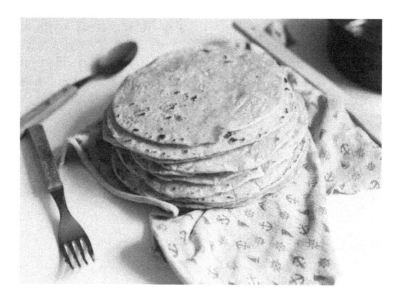

Around 450 BC, the Romans invented a more advanced form of milling than anything that had gone before: the process of water-milling. It is this process that resulted in breads that looked a lot whiter than historically present.

Along with the shocking white color came the status symbol that those who could afford water-milled bread had to be of the well-educated and wealthy classes.

As time progressed, those who were poor could only afford rye, bran, and coarser breads.

This is quite a paradox when we compare what people of today prefer, as well as their costs; the roles have been reversed. White bread is now considered a cheap and poor form of nutrition.

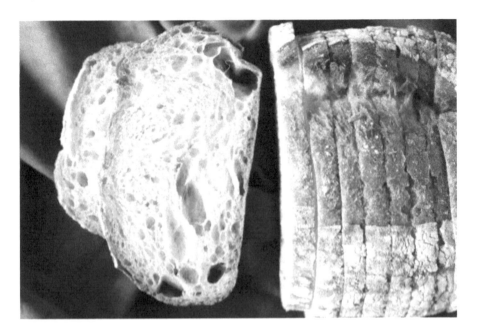

It was not until we hit the 19th century, more specifically 1834, that the steel-rolling mill started becoming the tool of choice to 'split' grains. Invented in Switzerland, the steel-roller mill moved away from crushing grains and towards breaking the grains open. This made it a lot simpler to separate the bran, endosperm, and germ from each other. It is because of this ability to split the constituents of grain that the gluten-intolerant individuals are super thankful. However, like many things that have a long history, there is a constant human desire to improve everything. With this in mind, the addition of chemicals came into play in the 20th century. With these additions, the bread produced became one step closer to how we know it today. The bread started to last much longer, had a softer texture, and had an amazing white appearance. The flour that was used was processed to an extent that essential minerals and vitamins were lost, leading to the standard operating procedures including flour enrichment within their processes.

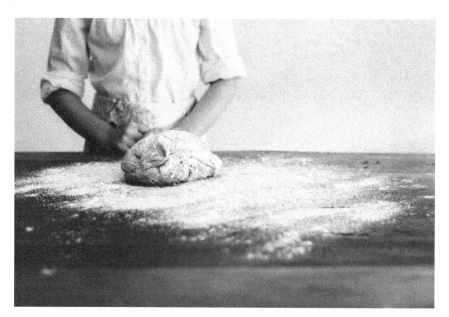

There are many individuals who think bread is made 100% from wheat. With that being said, bread can actually be made from any type of grain. Corn, barley, rice, rye, and whole wheat are but just a few of these variations. This does not mean that there will be no wheat when you are baking bread, seeing as wheat is an essential chemical component in the baking process. Wheat contains gluten that is vital to enable a loaf of bread to rise effectively. Without it, you will most probably need to get used to flatbreads, much like those kinds of breads for the gluten intolerant.

Now that we have established the different types of breads, how did we as the human race, get from the prehistoric flatbread to the fluffy loaf we all know so well? This was achieved due to three primary innovations, which include leavening, refined flour, and mechanized slicing. Leavening is the effect of making the bread rise so it can ultimately become light and fluffy. We refer to leavening agents, with the most common being that of yeast. Typically, we add a sachet of yeast to our dough, but historically, they would leave the bread open and exposed. Chemically, the process includes the yeast eating the sugars present in the grain. This is followed by the excretion of carbon dioxide that aerates the bread to its light and fluffy state.

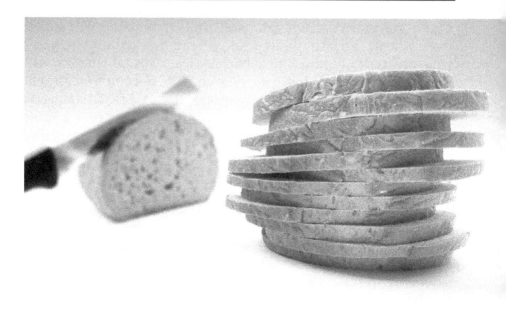

With the earliest bread grains being ground by hand and with rocks, we can reiterate that coarse and whole-grain bread like that of the pumpernickel, were bound to be the result of the historical methods used. The process of milling, as we discussed above, falls into this category, along with the sifting of flour to remove the bran and the bleaching of the flour itself to get that sparklingly white color that was desired.

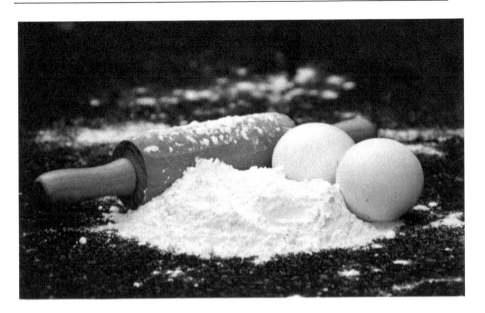

We walk through supermarkets and see the mechanized bread slicers that allow us to take our bread and cut it into equal slices. These machines have their initial origins in the year 1917 and were invented by the jeweler Otto Rohwedder. Many houses adopted the mechanized slicing technology, and the thickness of the received slice would go a long way to identifying the recipients' social class. The workers, gardeners, and cleaners would receive thick slices of bread with large amounts of crust, as well as the offcuts from the loaf. Seeing as these offcuts were given to those of poor wealth; the equal, pearly white slices with minimal hard crust were kept for the house owners, symbolizing their superiority and wealth.

Baking Bread in a Bread Machine

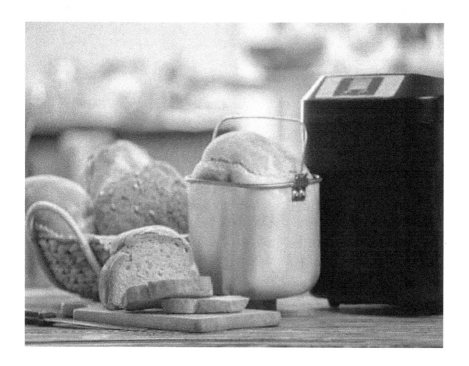

Bread Machine Cycles and Settings

The following are various cycles and settings that you can find on your bread machine:

1. Basic: This is ideal for basic American bread recipes. The setting is perfect for most savory yeast bread, but you can't use this cycle to make sweet yeast bread.

2. Sweet: This cycle is designed to make sweet yeast bread. Do not mix it with a quick bread cycle because quick bread does not contain yeast. This is the reason they bake at a different pace.

3. Whole Wheat: It takes more time to bake bread with whole wheat flour. Whole wheat means a longer rise time for any whole wheat baking using this setting.
4. French: This setting is used to make French bread and also used for other European-style bread. The temperature settings may vary slightly, and the timing is a bit longer on most machines.
5. Gluten-Free: People who follow gluten-free diets need gluten-free bread. This cycle is perfect for gluten-free bread. You can use gluten-free flours like coconut, almond, sorghum, or millet.
6. Quick/Rapid: Use this cycle if you are in a hurry. Depending on the machine, the cycle varies, but the shortening of rising times is common with this setting. You may need to use rapid rise yeast with some machines.
7. Quick Bread: This cycle is designed to use with quick bread recipes. Quick bread requires no rise time and can be baked immediately.
8. Jam: If you want to make homemade fruit spreads, then this cycle is for you. Cut your fruit into cubes for the best results. Do not puree in advance.
9. Dough: If you want to shape the loaves yourself, then use this cycle. This cycle does all the mixing and kneading and saves you time. The timer makes it easy to use. You can use this cycle to make pie crust, cookie dough, and other dough.
10. Time-Bake or Delayed Cycle: Some bread machines have this cycle. You add everything into the bread machine, then program it to start baking at a certain time.
11. Crust Functionality: You can select what type of crust you want with this function. Usually, there are three settings: soft, medium, and dark.
12. Other/Custom: Some machines have functions to create custom cycles. You can set up your own baking options and get the perfect loaf.

Remember, do not exceed your bread machine's capacity for a certain setting. Read the bread machine manual first before using it.

Everything About Gluten

Gluten is a group of families of storage proteins. They are naturally found in cereal grains such as barley, wheat, and rye. Gluten is not a health risk for most of the population. However, people with celiac disease cannot tolerate gluten.

Foods That Contain Gluten

- Grains: Barley, wheat bran, whole wheat, triticale, rye, spelt, farro, couscous, Kamut, bulgur, semolina, einkorn, farina, cracked wheat, wheat germ, durum, matzo, and mir.
- Products made from the above grains

You activate gluten molecules when you moisten the flour, then mix or knead it. Gluten is extremely important in baking because it gives traditional baked goods structure. Flour with a high protein (gluten) content (such as bread flour) will give you baked goods that are chewy and sturdy. On the other hand, flour with low protein content (such as cake flour) will give you baked goods that are light and tender.

Main Ingredients Used in Bread Making

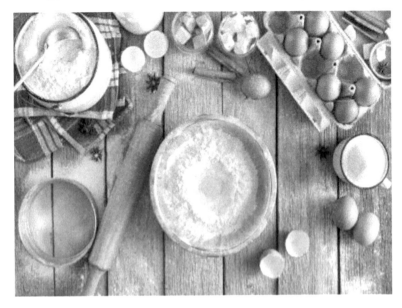

1. Flour: This is the main ingredient of bread. When baking bread, you need to use strong flour. Wheat flour is used in most bread products. Bread made with whole wheat grains/flour has a coarse texture and a rich flavor.

2. Water: Water is commonly used when baking bread. Water moistens the flour and helps form the dough. Water moistens the insoluble proteins and binds all the bread ingredients and produces a dough.

3. Yeast: Natural sugars are present in the flour. Yeast changes this sugar into minuscule bubbles of carbon dioxide that are trapped in the dough. When you bake, these bubbles expand and give the bread texture and lightness. Depending on your machine, you need to choose dry yeast or bread machine yeast.

4. Salt: Salt controls the action of the yeast. Salt gives stability to gluten; it improves flavor, controls the rate of fermentation, retains moisture, and affects the crust color and crumbs.

5. Sugar: Sugar acts as a food for yeast. It also improves the crust color and helps the bread retain moisture. You can use other ingredients such as maple syrup, honey, brown sugar, molasses, and corn syrup.
6. Milk: Milk makes the bread whiter, softer, provides moisture and a distinct flavor. Milk is usually used in skimmed and powdered form.
7. Eggs: Eggs give richness, lightness, and color to the bread. They also help the bread rise.
8. Oil, fat, butter, and lard: They provide flavor and softness to the bread. Fats and oils increase the nutritious value of the bread. It softens the crust and the crumbs and reduces elasticity. They help retain moisture and give flavor.

Preparing and Measuring Your Ingredients

Using the right type of flour
When choosing flour for your baking, you need to consider two things: quality and protein content.
Quality: Some companies use chemicals, so the flour looks white. Choose a company that doesn't use chemicals.
Protein content: The higher the protein, the "stronger" the flour. Choosing the right flour is important. Let's discuss different types of flours:

- All-purpose flour: 11.7% protein. You can use it in any recipe, but it is ideal for pie crust, quick bread, muffins, and cookies.
- Bread flour: 12.7% protein. With higher protein content, you will get a higher rise. So, use this bread for all your yeast baking, such as bagels, sandwich loaves, and pizza dough.
- White whole wheat flour: 13% protein. This flour's nutritional profile is similar to wheat flour but different in flavor and color. The flour acts like all-purpose flour.

- Whole wheat flour: 14% protein. This flour has more nutrition and robust flavor. You can bake whole wheat sandwich bread with it. To make other baked goods, start by replacing 25% of the flour, then increase as you get more experience.
- Self-rising flour: 8.5%. This flour is best for pancakes, scones, and biscuits.
- Italian-style flour: 8.5% protein. This is a low protein flour. It is best for flatbreads, thin-crust pizza, and focaccia.

Using the right yeast for the bread machine

Read the bread machine instructions to know what sort of yeast is recommended. The common types are bread machine yeast, rapid rise yeast, instant dry yeast, and active dry yeast.

- Bread machine yeast: It is specially made for bread machines. You can directly add it to the dry ingredients in your machine.
- Rapid rise yeast: Many bread machines have a quick/rapid cycle. You can use this yeast with a quick/rapid cycle.
- Instant dry yeast: It is a lot like rapid rise yeast.
- Active dry yeast: Usually, you need to dissolve the active dry yeast in water before using it. However, you can use it in some types of bread machines without proofing.

Top Bread Machine Tips

- You must read your bread machine's manual and understand how it works.
- Do not exceed the capacity of your bread machine pan. Even one teaspoon could make a difference.
- Check your bread machine's instructions to know the proper order.

- Use "bread machine bread flour" for the best result. It is the same thing as bread flour.
- Use room-temperature eggs.
- Do not use a delayed mix cycle when using milk
- Cut margarine or butter into small pieces before adding them into the machine.

High Altitude Baking

High altitude baking can be difficult. Anyone who lives 3,000 feet above the sea level understands the challenge. Here are tips on improving your high-altitude bread machine baking:

1. Moisture: You can change your source of moisture. Add one or two teaspoons of olive oil or use unsweetened applesauce, so the dough stays moist.
2. Increase moisture: Depending on your climate and altitude, you may need to add 2 to 4 tablespoons of more liquid (milk, buttermilk, water, etc.) per cup of flour.
3. Salt: Do not remove salt from your recipes. Use sea salt if you do not want excess sodium.
4. Lower sugar or yeast: If you are still not getting perfect bread, then lower the yeast. Cut it by 1/8 to ¼ of a teaspoon. Lower sugar amount by 1 to 2 teaspoons.
5. Liquid temperature: Using ice water instead of warm water will help. Remember, this method will not work if your bread machine has a preheat setting.
6. Adjust: You can adjust the baking time to get the result you are looking for.
7. Shrink: If everything fails, then shrink the loaf size. Smaller loaves do well at higher altitudes.

Troubleshooting
Small and heavy loaf

- Check measurements. Make sure flour and the liquid ratio is exact
- Make sure you are using fresh yeast

- Check dough consistency during the kneading cycle. You may need to add more flour or liquid
- Ingredients were added in the wrong order
- Too much whole grain or whole grain flour
- Too much dried fruit or other ingredients, such as nuts
- If the dough is too dry, then add one teaspoon of water at a time during the kneading cycle

Collapsed loaf

- Make sure you use a proper size pan for the recipe
- Check measurements (flour to liquid)
- During the kneading cycle, check dough consistency
- Do not use more yeast
- Add salt according to recipe recommendation
- If the weather is humid or warm, then
- Try rapid cycle
- Use refrigerated liquids
- Or bake during the coolest part of the day

Gummy texture—avoid underbaking

- Make sure you are using a large enough baking pan
- Use the right setting
- Use a darker setting if your machine has this option

Mushroom-shaped loaf

- Make sure the pan is large enough for the recipe
- Check measurements
- Too much yeast or water
- Too much sugar or too many sweet ingredients
- The bread pan is too small
- During the kneading cycle, check consistency
- If the weather is warm, then follow the collapsed loaf tips

Open, holey texture

- Check measurements
- Check consistency (during kneading cycle)
- Avoid using more yeast
- Add salt as described
- If the weather is warm, then use collapsed loaf tips

Very dense texture /bumpy, uneven top
- Measure flour lightly
- Do not use too much flour
- Check dough consistency during kneading

Underdone or burned
- Bread with a lot of milk and sugar brown faster
- Try adjusting the temperature

Crust too brown
- Use a lighter setting
- Remove loaf a few minutes before baking time

Overflowed
- Not enough salt—do not add more or less
- Check the type or amount of yeast
- Add 1 to 2 tablespoons of flour or adjust yeast by ¼ teaspoon
- Check if the water temperature is correct

No rise
- Yeast is old or low quality
- Measurement is wrong
- Flour has low protein/gluten content
- Salt measurement is wrong
- Salt came into contact with the yeast

Too much rise
- Too much yeast
- Too little salt
- Water temperature is incorrect
- The bucket is too small

Crust too thick
- Bread is left in the machine after the baking cycle is complete
- Flour has too little protein/gluten

Crust too light
- Crust setting is too light
- Too little sugar
- Recipe size is too large for the bucket

Bread-Machine Secrets You Need to Know

1. Start simple. If you are a beginner bread maker, then start with simple recipes. For example, choose pizza dough and/or focaccia.
2. Be careful about substitutions. Substituting whole wheat flour for all-purpose flour or white flour is not easy. As a beginner, strictly follow the recipes. Once you have a year of baking experience, then you can start experimenting. The same goes for the yeast. Different types of yeast will produce different results, so do not substitute.
3. You can open the lid. Check the dough after five minutes of adding the ingredients. You may notice various things, such as
- You forgot to attach the blade
- The dough is too moist. You need to add one tablespoon of flour at a time to fix it
- The dough is too dry—you need to add one tablespoon of water at a time to fix it
4. Know in which order you need to add ingredients in the machine. With most bread machines, you start with liquids then finish with dry ingredients.
5. Know the capacity of your machine.
6. You can use the basic cycle for most bread.
7. Use applesauce instead of butter or oil if you want a low-fat bread.
8. Yeast needs sugar, so use real sugar or honey or molasses.
9. Never place the yeast in direct contact with sugar or salt. Create a shallow pocket in the top of the flour with a spoon and place the yeast there. Make sure the yeast doesn't come into contact with the liquid by placing it in a shallow well at the top of the ingredients.
10. Use a whisk to aerate the flour. Then scoop the flour lightly into a dry measuring cup.

How to Store Your Bread

1. Storing bread dough: Prepare your dough according to the recipe. Allow rising. Then wrap it in a plastic wrap and place it in a plastic container or bag.

-   You can refrigerate bread dough for three to four days
-   You can freeze bread dough for up to one month

2. Where you slice matters: If you slice your bread at one end, then you will get an open-end moisture "leaking" problem. So, slice the loaf in half down the middle, cut servings from the loaves, and then press the loaves back together before storing. This will prevent leaking moisture problems.
3. Wrapping bread in foil or plastic instead of cloth keeps the soft bread longer.
4. If you want to preserve crispy crust, store large crusty loaves on the counter (unwrapped and cut-side down) at room temperature for a day or so.
5. For long-term storage (more than two days), wrap your bread in single-day portions and freeze. Thaw and reheat servings before serving.
6. Breadbox: A large breadbox will give you air circulation and balance humidity to store your bread properly. Do not wrap the bread in paper and then place it in the bread box.
7. Do not refrigerate: Do not keep your homemade bread in the refrigerator because it will stale quickly. However, you can put store-bought bread in the refrigerator.
8. Bread with added fat such as brioche and challah will take longer to stale. On the other hand, low-fat bread like baguettes will stale quickly.

Pro Tips to Make Perfect Bread

Whether you're just baking bread for the first time or you just want to bake better goodies, this section will give you all kinds of helpful insight to ensure that you make the most of your baking. From important elements to quick fixes and even simple basics, you'll find it all here.

Measurements Make a Difference

When it comes to baking, measurements are not merely a suggestion. Rather, they are a science. You have to be very careful about measuring out your ingredients. For starters, make sure that you go to a kitchen store or shop online to supply your kitchen with actual measuring tools. Make sure that you have liquid and dry measuring tools in various sizes.

The biggest mistakes that you want to avoid include:

Don't use liquid measures for dry ingredients, and vice versa

Tbsp and Tsp are interchangeable for liquid and dry. Cups, however, are not. If you need two cups of water, it needs to be two liquid cups. Don't believe there's a difference? Use a dry cup measure and fill it with water. Then, pour it into your liquid measuring cup. You'll quickly see that the measurement is less than exact.

Don't skip the salt!

Unless you are specifically altering a recipe for sodium content (in which case you should find a low or no-sodium version), salt is an ingredient for a reason, and you cannot leave it out. Even if it seems like it wouldn't make a difference, it could ruin a recipe.

Get a conversion chart, app, or magnet for the fridge

There are plenty of kitchen conversion guides out there that you can keep on hand. That way, if you need to convert measurements or make substitutions, you know exactly how to do it. You'll find all of your cooking and baking to be more enjoyable when you have conversions and substitutions at hand at all times.

If you're still in the beginner stages, you'll want to stick to the book as best as you can until you get the hang of things. Once you branch out and start to experiment, you can toss these rules out the window (except the liquid/dry measure one). The deliciousness of baking is in the details, and you cannot afford to make simple mistakes when it comes to measurements. There is a reason for the recipe, so if you want to get the best result, follow the instructions to the letter.

Quality Matters

When you are baking anything, the quality of the ingredients that you use will make a difference. It isn't to say that the store brand flour isn't as good as the name brand because it very well might be. However, you should be careful in choosing a higher-quality ingredient in order to get better results. If you have the choice, go to a baker's supply or a local bakery outlet to buy the good stuff at better prices. If not, make sure that you get to know your basic ingredients and which ones are best.

The more familiar you get with your own baking abilities and preferences, the more you will be able to decide for yourself where quality matters most. Until then, keep these tips in mind. Also, remember that higher protein content counts with your flour if you're baking bread. More protein means stronger gluten, which makes better bread. Cake flour has a softer texture and lower protein count, which makes it ideal for baking cakes and other desserts.

Recipes All Have a Reason

A lot of people prefer just to "throw in" the ingredients or measure hastily, which is fine if you're an expert or you're baking something that you've made 100 times before. If, however, you are trying to replicate something out of a recipe book, you need to follow the recipe. Even a single missed ingredient or mismeasurement can turn your bread into something completely different than what you wanted.

It's not like you are going to ruin everything by taking on baking with reckless abandon. If you're new at the bread machine game, though, you should get used to what you're doing before you throw caution to the wind and throw the recipe aside once you remind yourself of the baking temperature.

Even if you concoct your own recipes over time, you'll want to write down at least a rough estimate of what the measurement is. It's hard to share recipes that don't have finite measurements. While you might know exactly how much a "little" salt is, other people can't measure that accurately. Cooking takes skill, but baking is a science, and it should be treated as such.

Check Your Settings

Again, the process is important. In that, you should also be sure that you check the settings of your bread machine before you start any new baking program. Even if you think you left it on the right setting or programmed the right feature, you need to double-check every time. There is nothing worse than waiting an entire hour to realize that you've been using the wrong setting. At that point, your recipe will most likely be ruined.

For beginners, the pre-programmed settings should be perfect, for the most part. There are a lot more options for those who are more experienced with bread machines like the bread machine, and everyone will get there eventually. When in doubt, use the programs and features on the machine, and let it make the hard decisions for you. You'll get great results, and if the program isn't exactly right, you'll at least have a starting point to begin making adjustments.

Buttermilk Basics

Some people might not even understand exactly what buttermilk is. You don't have to be embarrassed; a lot of people don't know what this weird baking ingredient is for. Buttermilk, traditionally, was what was left after the cream was churned into butter. Most of the buttermilk that you find on the shelves today is cultured or made.

Buttermilk is used because it adds a slight tang to baked goods. It also increases the rise of the bread or pastry by reacting with the baking soda in the recipe. Buttermilk is in a lot of bread and dessert recipes. However, not everyone just happens to keep buttermilk around. If you aren't in the habit of keeping it around, or if you decide to bake something at the last minute, there is a solution. You can take a liquid measuring cup (one cup is fine). In a measuring cup, add a tbsp of lemon juice in the. Next, add milk up to half cup mark. Allow it to sit for a little bit, and voila, you have homemade buttermilk.

Try Something New

Experimenting is good. If you're a novice at baking bread or just starting to learn your bread machine, you might not want to stray too far from the traditional. However, if you are willing to make mistakes for the sake of success, experiment away! As you get more experienced in baking bread with your bread machine, you will be more comfortable in changing things up and seeing what all you can make on your own.

You can try ingredient substitutions, such as the common use of applesauce as a sweetener in baked goods. You can add ingredients to existing recipes, change baking times and temperatures, and even try and create your own great recipes using your bread machine.

Consistency Checks

The big difference with baking bread, compared to other cooking, is that you need to keep an eye on the consistency. While the good old "lightly brown" rule does stand in most cases, the consistency can be very different in a bread machine like the bread machine. Make sure that you capitalize on that "pause" feature and give yourself the chance to check in on your baked goods from time to time to ensure that they turn out their best.

You don't need to interrupt your baking processes too often. One should be enough. When you're making bread, it's a great idea to pause to remove the paddle, and at the same time, check on the bread and see how it's coming along. Not only does that allow you to ensure that the consistency is right, but it also allows you to get that paddle out before it's baked into the loaf and becomes a chore to remove.

How to Maintain Sourdough Starter

A sourdough starter is the "sour" in sourdough. It's a combination of flour, liquid, and yeast stored in a loosely covered jar or crock in the refrigerator. Frequent use or regular feeding keeps it alive. Some starters have been known to survive for generations!

There are probably as many sourdough starter recipes as there are wrinkles on an elephant. We won't go into them here; for now, we'd like to offer a few tips and facts for maintaining a sourdough starter.

Using A Starter

Bring refrigerated starter to room temperature before using it. You can place it in a bowl of warm water if you're in a hurry, or you can leave it out overnight if you plan to use it in the morning.

Like most things in life, the sourdough starter gets better with age. So, don't be discouraged if your first bread doesn't quite live up to your sourest expectations. Just keep baking with it, and very soon, you'll notice it taking on its tangy personality.

Experiment. Use your sourdough starter in some of your favorite recipes. Rye bread is incredibly yummy when soured. If your starter is roughly half liquid and half flour, when you add starter to a recipe, consider half the starter amount used as liquid and reduce the liquid in the recipe by that amount. If you choose to add 1 cup sourdough starter to a rye bread recipe that lists 1¼ cups water, count the 1 cup starter as ½ cup liquid and deduct that amount from your 1¼ cups water. For that recipe, your liquids would be 1 cup sourdough starter and ¾ cup water.

Maintaining A Starter

After each use, the starter needs to be replenished with equal amounts of liquid and flour. Please do so, then cover it loosely and leave it out at room temperature for several hours until it increases and turns spongy-looking. Stir it down, then refrigerate.

Your starter should always be kept in the refrigerator or freezer. The exceptions, for those first few days as it's developing, the few hours before it's used, and the few hours after it's replenished or fed.

Feed your starter once a month if you are not using it. Add equal amounts of flour and warm liquid (90° to 100°F). Cover loosely and allow it to stand in a warm location (70° to 95°F) until it expands and turns spongy-looking. Stir it down and then place it in the refrigerator, loosely covered.

Remove the starter from its container every so often and give the container a good wash job in hot water.

Sourdough starter ages best when handled with tender, loving care. So, do remember to feed it. If you're going to be gone or know you won't be baking with your starter for an extended time, you can freeze it. When you choose to use it again, allow your starter to sit at room temperature for 24 hours to thaw out and return to life.

If you'd want to create a "backup" of your starter for safekeeping or share it with friends across the country, consider dehydrating some of it. Here's how:

Spoon enough starter on foam-type paper plates or large wax-paper—lined trays to coat the entire surface with a thin layer of starter. A thin coating will dry completely in approximately 24 hours. Once thoroughly dry, lift it off in large pieces and place it in a food processor, blender, or grain mill. Process briefly until coarsely ground.

Store and put in a glass jar or plastic bag someplace cool. When you are ready to rehydrate your dried starter, place ½ cup warm water (90° to 100°F) in a 1½-quart glass or ceramic container. Add ¼ cup ground starter and then ¼ cup flour. Stir well with a wooden spoon. Place the container in a warm location (between 75° and 95°F), and within several hours your starter should show signs of life with surface bubbles. At that point, add another ½ cup warm water and ½ cup more flour, stir, and allow the starter to feed overnight at room temperature before you use it or loosely cover it and store it in your refrigerator for later use.

If, after freezing or several weeks of nonuse, your starter looks a little sluggish and isn't displaying its usual bubbly personality, reserve 1 or 2 tablespoons of the starter in a separate bowl and pour the rest away. Thoroughly wash the container and place the reserved starter back into the clean container. Add 1 cup warm liquid (90° to 100°F) and 1 cup flour. Cover loosely and let it stand in a warm place (70° to 95°F) for several hours until bubbly and a clear liquid begins to form on top. You may be required to repeat it once or twice to bring it back to its bubbly, sour-smelling self again.

To maintain a 70° to 95°F temperature, place it in a warm location like an oven with a pilot light on, a warm kitchen, water heater's top, or refrigerator. During the day, put it in the sunshine, in a bowl filled with water set on a warming tray or directly on a heating pad.

Rye Bread

1. Basic Rye Bread

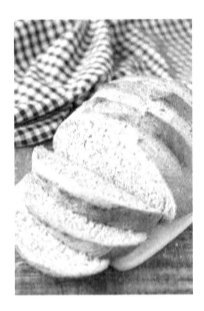

It is a simple rye bread prepared in the bread machine. For a better rise, more sugar is added.

Preparation time: 5 minutes

Cooking time: 3 hours

Servings: 12

Ingredients:

- 1 1/8 cups warm water
- 2 tbsps. molasses

- 1 tbsp. vegetable oil
- 1 tsp. salt
- 2 cups all-purpose flour
- 1 1/2 cups rye flour
- 3 tbsps. packed brown sugar
- 1 tbsp. unsweetened cocoa powder
- 3/4 tsp. caraway seed
- 2 tsp. bread machine yeast

Directions:

1. Assemble the ingredients as directed by your bread machine's manufacturer.
2. Then select the settings for whole wheat and light crust.

Nutrition:

Calories: 159

Carbohydrate: 32.5 g

Fat: 1.6 g

Protein: 3.6 g

2. Buttermilk Rye Bread

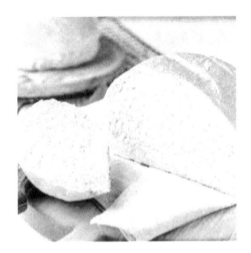

Buttermilk Rye Bread is lovely, and it makes beautiful toast, is fantastic in sandwiches, and is beautiful for an open face with turkey, chicken, and melted cheese.

Preparation time: 45 minutes

Cooking time: 1 hour & 15 minutes

Servings: 15

Ingredients:

- 1 1/3 cups water
- 2 tbsps. vegetable oil
- 2 tbsps. honey
- 1 1/2 tbsps. vinegar
- 2 tbsps. powdered buttermilk
- 2 1/3 cups bread flour
- 1 cup rye flour

- 1/3 cup dry potato flakes
- 1 tsp. salt
- 2 tsp. active dry yeast
- 1 tsp. caraway seed

Directions:

1. Add the ingredients following the order given by the machine's manufacturer into the bread machine pan.
2. Then set the machine to the setting for Basic or White Bread and push the start button.

Nutrition:

Calories: 59

Carbohydrate: 9.3 g

Fat: 2 g

Protein: 1.2 g

3. Caraway Rye Bread

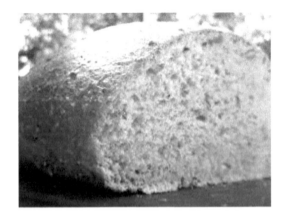

This light rye loaf is nicely flavored and has lots of caraway seeds. It's sweetened with molasses and brown sugar. Let to cool before cutting.

Preparation time: 10 minutes

Cooking time: 4 hours & 10 minutes

Servings: 12

Ingredients:

- 1 1/4 cups lukewarm water (100 degrees F/38 degrees C)
- 2 tbsps. dry milk powder
- 1 tsp. salt
- 2 tbsps. brown sugar
- 2 tbsps. molasses
- 2 tbsps. butter
- 3/4 cup whole wheat flour

- 1 3/4 cups bread flour
- 3/4 cup rye flour
- 1 1/2 tbsps. caraway seeds
- 1 3/4 tsp. active dry yeast

Directions:

1. In the bread machine pan, add water at room temperature, milk powder, salt, brown sugar, molasses, butter, whole wheat flour, bread flour, rye flour, caraway seeds, and yeast.

2. Then set the machine to the setting for Basic or White Bread and push the start button.

Nutrition:

Calories: 93

Carbohydrate: 16.5 g

Fat: 2.3 g

Protein: 2.4 g

4. Chai Cake

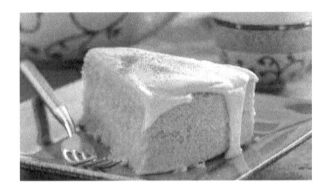

It isn't exactly a coffee cake but rather a bread machine cake that is very moist. This bread turned out to be great in the morning or as a snack/dessert. You can top your slices with strawberry cream cheese, although you can top with anything to satisfy your sweet tooth.

Preparation time: 15 minutes

Cooking time: 3 hours & 55 minutes

Servings: 10

Ingredients:

- 1 (1.1 oz) package chai tea powder
- 3/4 cup hot water
- 1/4 cup Chardonnay wine
- 1/2 tsp. vanilla extract
- 1 egg yolk
- 1/2 cup frozen unsweetened raspberries
- 1 tbsp. butter, room temperature

- 1/2 cup bread flour
- 1/4 cup rye flour
- 1 cup all-purpose flour
- 1/2 cup wheat bran
- 1 (.25 oz.) package active dry yeast
- 1/2 cup coarsely chopped walnuts
- 1/2 tsp. caraway seed
- 1/4 cup white sugar
- 1 tsp. coarse smoked salt flakes

Directions:

1. Use 1 packet or 2 tbsp of dry mix mixed into 3/4 cup of hot water to make the chai tea. Let to cool for around ten 10 minutes.

2. Into bread machine pan, mix the chai tea, Chardonnay, vanilla extract, egg yolk, frozen raspberries, and butter. Then pour in bread flour, rye flour, all-purpose flour, wheat bran, yeast, walnuts, caraway seed, sugar, and salt.

3. Set machine to "Sweet" setting with a "Light Crust" and press the start button. Once bread finishes baking, let it cool for a minimum of half an hour before slicing. Serve.

Nutrition:

Calories: 184

Carbohydrate: 27.9 g

Fat: 6.3 g   **Protein:** 4.3 g

5. Danish Rugbrod

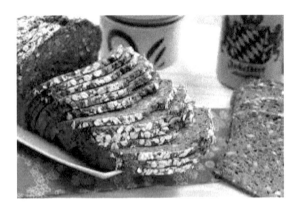

Danish Rugbrod bread is made from a very spongy dough. The rye gives it a unique texture and the butter an impressive bite.

Preparation time: 10 minutes

Cooking time: 3 hours & 10 minutes

Servings: 24

Ingredients:

- 1 1/2 cups water
- 1 tbsp. honey
- 1 tbsp. butter
- 1 tsp. salt
- 2 cups rye flour
- 1 cup all-purpose flour
- 1 cup whole wheat flour
- 1/4 cup rye flakes (optional)
- 1 tbsp. white sugar

- 2 tsp. bread machine yeast

Directions:

1. Into the bread machine pan, add the following in this order: water, honey, butter, salt, rye flour, all-purpose flour, whole wheat flour, rye flakes, sugar, and yeast.

2. Set the machine to the setting for basic and start it.

Nutrition:

Calories: 80

Carbohydrate: 16.5 g

Fat: 0.8 g

Protein: 2.2 g

6. Danish Spiced Rye Bread

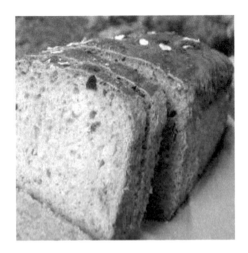

An old-fashioned Danish rye bread that is made easy by using the bread machine. This highly spiced bread is excellent with Danish open-faced sandwiches (smorrebrod) and mostly served on a Christmas holiday. It's perfect for individuals who love a spiced twist to their bread.

Preparation time: 20 minutes

Cooking time: 3 hours & 25 minutes

Servings: 16

Ingredients:

- 1 cup milk
- 1 cup of water
- 3 tbsps. butter
- 1/2 cup light molasses
- 1/3 cup white sugar

- 1 tbsp. grated orange zest
- 1 tbsp. fennel seed
- 1 tbsp. anise seed
- 1 tbsp. caraway seed
- 1 tbsp. cardamom
- 1 tsp. salt
- 2 (.25 oz.) packages active dry yeast
- 1/4 cup warm water at 110 F
- 2 cups rye flour
- 5 cups all-purpose flour
- 3 tbsps. butter, melted

Directions:

1. Warm milk in a medium saucepan until it's scalding and small bubbles form around the edges, and just before the milk starts to boil.

2. Remove the pan from the heat source and mix in the caraway seed, water, orange zest, butter, salt, molasses, cardamom, sugar, and anise seed. Let to step and cool for half an hour at lukewarm.

3. Mix the warm water and the yeast in a bread maker and then leave to stand for 5 minutes. Add the spice mixture and cooled milk into the bread machine containing the yeast mixture.

4. Pour the flour into the bread machine. Set to dough cycle and then run it. Coat two 9x5 inch loaf pans with grease.

5. Once the dough cycle is done, take out the dough from the machine, separate it in half, shape into two loaves, and then transfer to the loaf pans prepared.

6. Cover loaves and rise within 30 minutes or until a small dent is formed on the loaves when you poke with your finger.

7. Warm oven to 375 F, then bake within 35 to 40 minutes until the loaves sound hollow once tapped at the bottom. Use melted butter to rub the hot loaves and then let to cool before serving.

Nutrition:

Calories: 287

Carbohydrate: 53.5 g

Fat: 5.5 g

Protein: 6.4 g

7. Health Dynamics Rye Bread

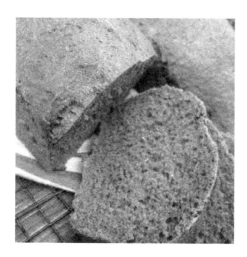

The use of rye flour is evident in the crackling crisp crumb, the pleasant mild sour tang, and the unyielding firmness. It is bread for people who like to put their teeth into a long, chewy mouthful.

Preparation time: 15 minutes

Cooking time: 46 minutes

Servings: 12

Ingredients:

- 2 eggs
- 3/4 cup warm water
- 2 tbsps. vegetable oil
- 2 tbsps. molasses
- 2 1/2 cups rye flour
- 1/4 cup cornstarch

- 2 tsp. lecithin
- 1 1/4 tsp. sea salt
- 3 tsp. active dry yeast

Directions:

1. Into the bread machine pan, put the ingredients in the order suggested by the manufacturer. Set the machine to the setting for Regular cycle and medium crust and push Start.

2. Check the consistency of the dough as it mixes. It should be a little bit sticky.

Nutrition:

Calories: 136

Carbohydrate: 21.8 g

Fat: 4.3 g

Protein: 3.4 g

8. Montana Russian Black Bread

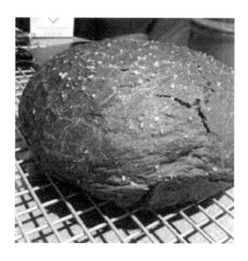

It is a very flavorful and healthy bread, and a little goes a long way. You'll want to serve it with lots of butter!

Preparation time: 20 minutes

Cooking time: 3 hours & 35 minutes

Servings: 10

Ingredients:

- 2 1/2 cups whole wheat bread flour
- 1 cup rye flour
- 3 tbsps. unsweetened cocoa powder
- 2 tbsps. bread flour
- 1 tbsp. wheat germ
- 1 tbsp. caraway seeds
- 2 tsp. active dry yeast
- 1 cup flat warm porter beer

- 1/2 cup strong brewed coffee
- 2 tbsps. balsamic vinegar
- 2 tbsps. olive oil
- 2 tbsps. honey
- 1 tbsp. molasses
- 1 tsp. sea salt
- 1/4 tsp. onion powder
- 1 egg white
- 1 tbsp. warm water

Directions:

1. In the bread machine, put in the whole wheat bread flour, rye flour, cocoa powder, bread flour, wheat germ, caraway seeds, yeast, beer, coffee, vinegar, olive oil, honey, molasses, sea salt, and onion powder, following the order of ingredients recommended by the manufacturer.

2. Choose the kneading cycle on the machine. Using your parchment paper to line the bottom of a baking sheet.

3. Take the dough out from the bread machine, place it onto the prepared baking sheet, form the dough into the shape of a rustic loaf.

4. Cut slits in a crisscross pattern on the top surface of the loaf. Allow the dough to rise in volume for 1 hour— Preheat the oven to 395°F (202°C).

5. In a small bowl, combine the warm water and egg white. Use a brush to coat the top of the loaf with the egg white mixture.

6. Put in the preheated oven and bake for 45-50 minutes until the bread is thoroughly cooked. Cool down for 1 hour before serving.

Nutrition:

Calories: 241

Carbohydrate: 41.4 g

Fat: 4.5 g

Protein: 8.3 g

9. Mustard Wheat Rye Sandwich Bread

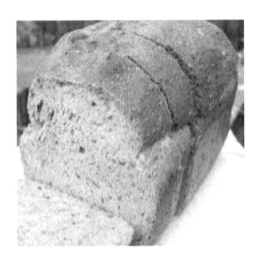

This sandwich bread is fantastic. It makes the perfect Rueben sandwich or grilled cheese! You can shape the bread in a circle and then bake free form in la cloche.

Preparation time: 5 minutes

Cooking time: 3 hours & 5 minutes

Servings: 12

Ingredients:

- 1 cup warm water at 110 F
- 1/2 cup Dijon-style prepared mustard
- 2 tbsps. olive oil
- 1 1/2 tbsps. molasses
- 2 cups unbleached all-purpose flour
- 2/3 cup rye flour

- 2/3 cup whole wheat flour
- 1 1/2 tbsps. vital wheat gluten
- 2 1/2 tsp. active dry yeast

Directions:

1. Into the bread machine pan, assemble all the ingredients according to the machine maker's instructions.
2. Then use the setting for basic or white bread and press start.

Nutrition:

Calories: 163

Carbohydrate: 29.9 g

Fat: 2.7 g

Protein: 4.5 g

10.   New York Rye Bread

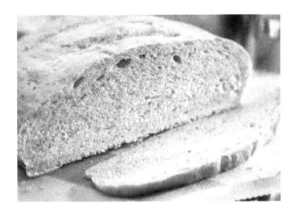

This bread has an intense rye flavor; it's traditionally baked in a bread machine. It's good with corned beef, pastrami, or sauerkraut.

Preparation time: 5 minutes

Cooking time: 3 hours & 5 minutes

Servings: 12

Ingredients:

- 1 1/8 cups warm water
- 1 1/3 tbsps. vegetable oil
- 2 tbsps. honey
- 1 tsp. salt
- 2 2/3 tsp. caraway seed
- 1 1/3 cups rye flour
- 2 1/3 cups bread flour
- 1/4 cup vital wheat gluten

- 1/4 cup dry milk powder
- 2 1/2 tsp. active dry yeast

Directions:

1. Put all the ingredients as directed by your machine's manual into the bread machine.
2. Select the setting for cycle to Basic or White. Press start.

Nutrition:

Calories: 90

Carbohydrate: 14.8 g

Fat: 1.8 g

Protein: 3.9 g

Nut and Seed Breads

11.　　Flax and Sunflower Seed Bread

Preparation Time: 5 Minutes

Cooking Time: 25 Minutes

Servings: 8

Ingredients:

- 1 1/3 cups water
- Two tablespoons butter softened
- Three tablespoons honey
- 2/3 cups of bread flour
- One teaspoon salt
- One teaspoon active dry yeast
- 1/2 cup flax seeds
- 1/2 cup sunflower seeds

Directions:

1. With the manufacturer's suggested order, add all the ingredients (apart from sunflower seeds) to the bread machine's pan.
2. The select basic white cycle, then press start.
3. Just in the knead cycle that your machine signals alert sounds, add the sunflower seeds.

Nutrition:

Calories: 140

Cholesterol: 4

Sodium: 169

Protein: 4.2

Total Carbohydrate: 22.7

Total Fat: 4.2

12.   Honey and Flaxseed Bread

Preparation Time: 5 Minutes

Cooking Time: 25 Minutes

Servings: 8

Ingredients:

- 1 1/8 cups water
- 1 1/2 tablespoons flaxseed oil
- Three tablespoons honey
- 1/2 tablespoon liquid lecithin
- 3 cups whole wheat flour
- 1/2 cup flax seed
- Two tablespoons bread flour
- Three tablespoons whey powder
- 1 1/2 teaspoons sea salt
- Two teaspoons active dry yeast

Directions:

1. In the bread machine pan, put in all of the ingredients following the order recommended by the manufacturer.
2. Choose the Wheat cycle on the machine and press the Start button to run the machine.

Nutrition:

Calories: 174   **Total Carbohydrate:** 30.8

Sodium: 242   **Protein:** 7.1

Total Fat: 4.9   **Cholesterol:** 1

13. Pumpkin and Sunflower Seed Bread

Preparation Time: 5 Minutes

Cooking Time: 25 Minutes

Servings: 8

Ingredients:

- 1 (.25 ounce) package instant yeast
- 1 cup of warm water
- 1/4 cup honey
- Four teaspoons vegetable oil
- 3 cups whole wheat flour
- 1/4 cup wheat bran (optional)
- One teaspoon salt
- 1/3 cup sunflower seeds
- 1/3 cup shelled, toasted, chopped pumpkin seeds

Directions:

1. Into the bread machine, put the ingredients according to the order suggested by the manufacturer.
2. Next is setting the machine to the whole wheat setting, then press the start button.
3. You can add the pumpkin and sunflower seeds at the beep if your bread machine has a signal for nuts or fruit.

Nutrition:

Calories: 148

Total Carbohydrate: 24.1

 Cholesterol: 0

Protein: 5.1

Total Fat: 4.8

Sodium: 158

14.   Seven Grain Bread

Preparation Time: 5 Minutes

Cooking Time: 25 Minutes

Servings: 8

Ingredients:

- 1 1/3 cups warm water
- One tablespoon active dry yeast
- Three tablespoons dry milk powder
- Two tablespoons vegetable oil
- Two tablespoons honey
- Two teaspoons salt
- One egg
- 1 cup whole wheat flour
- 2 1/2 cups bread flour
- 3/4 cup 7-grain cereal

Directions:

1. Follow the order of putting the ingredients into the pan of the bread machine recommended by the manufacturer.

2. Choose the Whole Wheat Bread cycle on the machine and press the Start button to run the machine.

Nutrition:

Total Carbohydrate: 50.6

 Cholesterol: 24

Total Fat: 5.2

Sodium: 629

Protein:9.8

15.   **Wheat Bread with Flax Seed**

Preparation Time: 5 Minutes

Cooking Time: 25 Minutes

Servings: 8

Ingredients:

- 1 (.25 ounce) package active dry yeast
- 1 1/4 cups whole wheat flour
- 3/4 cup ground flax seed
- 1 cup bread flour
- One tablespoon vital wheat gluten
- Two tablespoons dry milk powder
- One teaspoon salt
- 1 1/2 tablespoons vegetable oil
- 1/4 cup honey
- 1 1/2 cups water

Directions:

1. In the bread machine pan, put the ingredients following the order recommendation of the manufacturer.
2. Then set the machine to the setting for Basic or White Bread and push the start button.

Nutrition:

Calories: 168 calories   **Total Carbohydrate:** 22.5

Cholesterol: 1   **Protein:** 5.5

Total Fat: 7.3

Sodium: 245

16.   High Fiber Bread

Preparation Time: 5 Minutes

Cooking Time: 25 Minutes

Servings: 8

Ingredients:

- 1 2/3 cups warm water
- Four teaspoons molasses
- One tablespoon active dry yeast
- 2 2/3 cups whole wheat flour
- 3/4 cup ground flax seed
- 2/3 cup bread flour
- 1/2 cup oat bran
- 1/3 cup rolled oats
- 1/3 cup amaranth seeds
- One teaspoon salt

Directions:

1. In the bread machine pan, put in the water, molasses, yeast, wheat flour, ground flaxseed, bread flour, oat bran, rolled oats, amaranth seeds, and salt in the manufacturer's suggested order of ingredients. Choose the Dough cycle on the machine and press the Start button; let the machine finish the whole Dough cycle.

2. Put the dough on a clean surface that is covered with a little bit of flour. Shape the dough into two loaves and put it on a baking stone. Use a slightly wet cloth to

shelter the loaves and allow it to rise in volume for about 1 hour until it has doubled in size.

3. Preheat the oven to 375°F.

4. Put in the warm-up oven and bake for 20-25 minutes until the top part of the loaf turns golden brown. Let the loaf slide onto a clean working surface and tap the loaf's bottom part gently. The bread is done if you hear a hollow sound when tapped.

Nutrition:

Calories: 101

Total Fat: 2.1

Sodium: 100

Total Carbohydrate: 18.2

Cholesterol: 0

Protein: 4

17.   High Flavor Bran Head

Preparation Time: 5 Minutes

Cooking Time: 25 Minutes

Servings: 8

Ingredients:

- 1 1/2 cups warm water
- Two tablespoons dry milk powder
- Two tablespoons vegetable oil
- Two tablespoons molasses
- Two tablespoons honey
- 1 1/2 teaspoons salt
- 2 1/4 cups whole wheat flour
- 1 1/4 cups bread flour
- 1 cup whole bran cereal
- Two teaspoons active dry yeast

Directions:

1. In the pan of your bread machine, move all the ingredients directed by the machine's maker.
2. Set the machine to either the whole grain or whole wheat setting. Press start.

Nutrition:

Calories: 146 calories   **Total Fat:** 2.4

Sodium: 254   **Total Carbohydrate:** 27.9

Cholesterol: 1

Protein: 4.6

18.   High Protein Bread

Preparation Time: 5 Minutes

Cooking Time: 25 Minutes

Servings: 8

Ingredients:

- Two teaspoons active dry yeast
- 1 cup bread flour
- 1 cup whole wheat flour
- 1/4 cup soy flour
- 1/4 cup powdered soy milk
- 1/4 cup oat bran
- One tablespoon canola oil
- One tablespoon honey
- One teaspoon salt
- 1 cup of water

Directions:

1. Into the bread machine's pan, put the ingredients by following the order suggested by the manufacturer.
2. Set the machine to either the regular setting or the basic medium.
3. Push the Start button.

Nutrition:

Calories: 137 calories   **Total Fat:** 2.4

Sodium: 235   **Total Carbohydrate:** 24.1

Cholesterol: 0   **Protein:** 6.5

19. Whole Wheat Bread with Sesame Seeds

Preparation Time: 5 Minutes

Cooking Time: 25 Minutes

Servings: 8

Ingredients:

- 1/2 cup water
- Two teaspoons honey
- One tablespoon vegetable oil
- 3/4 cup grated zucchini
- 3/4 cup whole wheat flour
- 2 cups bread flour
- One tablespoon chopped fresh basil
- Two teaspoons sesame seeds
- One teaspoon salt
- 1 1/2 teaspoons active dry yeast

Directions:

1. Follow the order of putting the ingredients into the bread machine pan recommended by the manufacturer.
2. Choose the Basic Bread cycle or the Normal setting on the machine.

Nutrition:

Calories: 153 calories   **Sodium:** 235

Total Carbohydrate: 28.3 **Cholesterol:** 0

Protein: 5   **Total Fat:** 2.3

20. Bagels with Poppy Seeds

Preparation Time: 5 Minutes

Cooking Time: 25 Minutes

Servings: 8

Ingredients:

- 1 cup of warm water
- 1 1/2 teaspoons salt
- Two tablespoons white sugar
- 3 cups bread flour
- 2 1/4 teaspoons active dry yeast
- 3 quarts boiling water
- Three tablespoons white sugar
- One tablespoon cornmeal
- One egg white
- Three tablespoons poppy seeds

Directions:

1. In the bread machine's pan, pour in the water, salt, sugar, flour, and yeast following the order of ingredients suggested by the manufacturer. Choose the Dough setting on the machine.

2. Once the machine has finished the whole cycle, place the dough on a clean surface covered with a little bit of flour; let it rest. While the dough is resting on the floured surface, put 3 quarts of water in a big pot and let it boil. Add in 3 tablespoons of sugar and mix.

3. Divide the dough evenly into nine portions and shape each into a small ball. Press down each dough ball until it is flat. Use your thumb to make a shack in the center of each flattened dough. Increase the hole's size in the center and smoothen out the dough around the hole area by spinning the dough on your thumb or finger. Use a clean cloth to cover the formed bagels and let it sit for 10 minutes.

4. Cover the bottom part of an ungreased baking sheet evenly with cornmeal. Place the bagels gently into the boiling water. Let it boil for 1 minute and flip it on the other side halfway through. Let the bagels drain quickly on a clean towel. Place the boiled bagels onto the prepared baking sheet. Coat the topmost of each bagel with egg white and top it off with your preferred toppings.

5. Put the bagels into the preheated 375°F (190°C) oven and bake for 20-25 minutes until it turns nice brown.

Nutrition:

Calories: 50 calories

Total Fat: 1.3

Sodium: 404

Total Carbohydrate: 8.8

Cholesterol: 0

Protein: 1.4

21. Bruce's Honey Sesame Bread

Preparation Time: 5 Minutes

Cooking Time: 25 Minutes

Servings: 8

Ingredients:

- 1 1/4 cups water
- 1/4 cup honey
- One tablespoon powdered buttermilk
- 1 1/2 teaspoons salt
- 3 cups bread flour
- Three tablespoons wheat bran
- 1/2 cup sesame seeds, toasted
- 2 1/4 teaspoons active dry yeast

Directions:

1. Into the bread machine's pan, place all the ingredients by following the order endorsed by your machine's manufacturer.

2. Then set the machine to the setting for Basic or White Bread and push the start button.

Nutrition:

Calories: 62 calories

Total Carbohydrate: 8.4

Cholesterol: 1

Protein: 1.7

Total Fat: 3.1   **Sodium:** 295

22.   Moroccan Ksra

Preparation Time: 5 Minutes

Cooking Time: 25 Minutes

Servings: 8

Ingredients:

- 7/8 cup water
- 2 1/4 cups bread flour
- 3/4 cup semolina flour
- One teaspoon anise seed
- 1 1/2 teaspoons salt
- 1/2 teaspoon white sugar
- Two teaspoons active dry yeast
- One tablespoon olive oil
- One tablespoon sesame seed

Directions:

1. In a bread machine, put the first set of ingredients according to the manufacturer's recommendation. Set to DOUGH cycle and select Start. In this procedure, refrain from mixing in the sesame seeds and olive oil.

2. When the dough cycle signal stops, take the dough from the machine and deflate by punching down. Cut the dough into two halves and form it into balls. Pat the balls into a 3/4-inch thickness. Put the flattened dough on a floured baking sheet. Cover the baking sheet with

towels and let it stand for about 30 minutes to rise to double.

3. Set the oven to 200 degrees C (400 degrees F) to preheat. Spread the top of the loaves with olive oil using a brush and garnish with sesame seeds, if preferred. Using a fork, puncture the top of each loaf all over.

4. Place the pans in the heated oven, then bake for 20 to 25 minutes, or until colors are golden and they sound hollow when tapped. Serve either warm or cold.

Nutrition:

Calories: 111 calories

Total Fat: 1.6

Sodium: 219

Total Carbohydrate: 20.2

Cholesterol: 0

Protein: 3.6

23. Bread Sticks with Sesame Seeds

Preparation Time: 5 Minutes

Cooking Time: 25 Minutes

Servings: 8

Ingredients:

- 1 1/3 cups warm water
- Three tablespoons butter softened
- 4 cups bread flour
- Two teaspoons salt
- 1/4 cup white sugar
- 1/4 cup sesame seeds
- Two tablespoons dry milk powder
- 2 1/2 teaspoons active dry yeast

Directions:

1. Into the bread machine pan, set the ingredients according to the order given by the manufacturer. Put the machine to the Dough cycle and then push the Start button. Use cooking spray to spritz two baking sheets.

2. Preheat the oven. After the dough cycle comes to an end, place the dough onto a lightly oiled surface. Separate the dough into 18 pieces. Fold every piece on a board oiled from the middle of the amount to the outside edges. It is to create breadsticks. Transfer the

breadsticks onto the prepared pans placing at least one inch apart.

3. Bake for around 15 minutes using the oven until golden. Transfer to a wire rack to cool.

Nutrition:

Calories: 154

Total Fat: 3.5

Sodium: 278

Total Carbohydrate: 26

Cholesterol: 5

Protein: 4.5

24.   Apricot Cake Bread

Preparation Time: 20 Minutes

Cooking Time: 4 Hours and 30 Minutes

Servings: 8

Ingredients:

- 2 cups water, lukewarm
- 1 large egg, at room temperature
- ¾ cup orange juice
- 2 tbsp. butter, unsalted, softened
- 1 cup dried apricots, snipped
- 2 cups all-purpose flour
- 1 cup sugar
- 2 tbsp. baking powder
- ¼ tsp. baking soda
- 1 tsp. salt
- ¾ cup chopped nuts

Directions:

1. Take a medium bowl, place apricots in it, pour in water, and let soak for 30 minutes.
2. Then remove apricots from the water, reserve the water, and chop apricots into pieces.
3. Gather the remaining ingredients needed for the bread.
4. Power on bread machine that has about 2 pounds of the bread pan.

5. Put all the ingredients into the bread machine pan, except for apricots and nuts in the order mentioned in the ingredients list.

6. Press the "Bread" button, press the start button, let mixture knead for 5 minutes, add chopped apricots and nuts and continue kneading for 5 minutes until all the pieces have thoroughly combined and incorporated.

7. Select the "basic/white" cycle, press the up/down arrow to do baking to 4 hours, choose light or medium color for the crust, and press the start button.

8. When the timer of the bread machine beeps, open the machine.

9. It should come out spotless, else bake for another 10 to 15 minutes.

10. Cut bread into eight slices and then serve.

Nutrition:

Calories: 144

Fat (g): 3.6

Protein (g): 3.9

Carbs: 25.6

25. Cherry and Almond Bread

Preparation Time: 10 Minutes

Cooking Time: 4 Hours

Servings: 8

Ingredients:

- 1 cup milk, lukewarm
- ½ cup butter, unsalted, softened
- 2 eggs, at room temperature
- 2 cups bread flour
- 6 oz. dried cherries
- 1 cup slivered almonds, toasted
- ½ tsp. salt
- 0.25 oz. dry yeast, active
- 1 cup sugar

Directions:

1. Gather all the ingredients needed for the bread.
2. Power on bread machine that has about 2 pounds of the bread pan.
3. Add all the ingredients in the order mentioned in the ingredients list into the bread machine pan.
4. Press the "Dough" button, key the left button, and let mixture knead for 5 to 10 minutes.
5. Then select the "basic/white" down arrow to set baking time to 4 hours, select light or medium color for the crust, and press the start button.

6. Then prudently lift out the bread and put it on a wire rack for 1 hour or more until cooled.

7. Cut bread into sixteen slices and then serve.

Nutrition:

Calories: 125

Fat (g): 3

Protein (g): 4

Carbs: 20.4

26. Nutty Wheat Bread

Preparation Time: 10 Minutes

Cooking Time: 4 Hours

Servings: 12

Ingredients:

- 1 cup water, lukewarm
- 2 tbsp. olive oil
- 2 tbsp. honey
- 2 tbsp. molasses
- 1 cup whole wheat flour
- 2 cups bread flour
- 2 ¼ tsp. dry yeast, active
- 1 ½ tsp. salt
- 1/3 cup chopped pecans
- 1/3 cup chopped walnuts

Directions:

1. Gather all the ingredients needed for the bread.
2. Power on bread machine that has about 2 pounds of the bread pan.
3. Add all the ingredients in the order listed in the ingredients list into the bread machine pan except for pecans and nuts.
4. Press the "Dough" switch, press the start button, let mixture knead for 5 minutes, add pecans and nuts, and then continue kneading for another 5 minutes until all

the ingredients have thoroughly combined and incorporated.

5. Then select the "basic/white" cycle, press the up/down arrow to make the baking time to 4 hours.

6. Select light or medium color for the crust, and press the start button.

7. Then put the bread on a wire rack for 1 hour or more until cooled.

8. Cut bread into twelve slices and then serve.

Nutrition:

Calories: 187

Fat (g): 7

Protein (g): 5

Carbs: 28

27.   Hazelnut Yeast Bread

Preparation Time: 10 Minutes

Cooking Time: 3 Hours

Servings: 16

Ingredients:

- 2/3 cup milk, lukewarm
- 2 tbsp. butter, unsalted, melted
- 1 egg, at room temperature
- ½ tsp. almond extract, unsweetened
- ½ tsp. salt
- 2 cups bread flour
- 2 tbsp. sugar
- 0.25 oz. dry yeast, active
- ½ cup chopped hazelnuts, toasted

Directions:

1. Gather all the ingredients needed for the bread.
2. Then power on bread machine that has about 2 pounds of the bread pan.
3. Add all the ingredients in the order stated in the ingredients list into the bread machine pan except for nuts.
4. Press the "Dough" button, press the start button, let mixture knead for 5 minutes, add nuts, and then knead for another 5 minutes until all the ingredients have thoroughly combined and incorporated.

5. Then select the "basic/white" cycle, or press the up/down arrow to set baking time to 3 hours.

6. Select light or medium color for the crust, and then press the start button.

7. Put it on a wire rack for 1 hour or more until cooled.

8. Cut bread into sixteen slices and then serve.

Nutrition:

Calories: 139

Fat (g): 6

Protein (g): 5

Carbs: 18

28.   **Date-Nut Yeast Bread**

Preparation Time: 10 Minutes

Cooking Time: 4 Hours

Servings: 12

Ingredients:

- 1 cup water, lukewarm
- 1 tbsp. butter, unsalted, softened
- 3 ¼ cups bread flour
- 0.5 oz. dry yeast, active
- 2 tbsp. brown sugar
- ½ tsp. salt
- ½ cup dates, chopped
- ¼ cup walnuts, chopped

Directions:

1. Gather all the ingredients needed for the bread.
2. Power on bread machine that has about 2 pounds of the bread pan.
3. Add all the ingredients in the order cited in the ingredients list into the bread machine pan.
4. Press the "Dough" button, push the start button.
5. Allow the mixture to knead for 5 to 10 minutes until all the pieces have been thoroughly combined and incorporated.
6. Select the "basic/white" cycle, or press the up/down arrow to set baking day to 4 hours.

7. Select light or medium color for the crust, and then press the start button.

8. Then handover it to a wire rack for one hour or more until cooled.

9. Cut bread into twelve slices and then serve.

Nutrition:

Calories: 123

Fat (g): 2

Protein (g): 4

Carbs: 24

29.   **Walnut Bread**

Preparation Time: 10 Minutes

Cooking Time: 4 Hours

Servings: 12

Ingredients:

- 1 ½ cups water, lukewarm
- 1 egg, at room temperature
- 4 tbsp. butter, unsalted, softened
- 3 cups bread flour
- 2 tbsp. dry yeast, active
- ½ cup dry milk powder, nonfat
- 3 tbsp. sugar
- 1 tbsp. salt
- 2 ½ cups chopped walnuts, toasted

Directions:

1. Gather all the ingredients needed for the bread.
2. Then power on bread machine that has about 2 pounds of the bread pan.
3. Add all the ingredients in the order revealed in the ingredients list into the bread machine pan.
4. Press the "Dough" button, press the start button, and let mixture knead for 5 to 10 minutes until all the ingredients have thoroughly combined and incorporated.

5. Select the "basic/white" cycle, key the up/down arrow to set baking time to 4 hours.

6. Select light or medium color for the crust, and press the start button.

7. Then sensibly lift out the bread, and put it on a wire rack for 1 hour or more until cooled.

8. Cut bread into twelve slices and then serve.

Nutrition:

Calories: 135

Fat (g): 5

Protein (g): 5

Carbs: 19

30.   Cranberry Walnut Bread

Preparation Time: 10 Minutes

Cooking Time: 4 Hours

Servings: 16

Ingredients:

- 1 ½ cups water, lukewarm
- 2 tsp. butter, unsalted, softened
- 3 cups bread flour
- ½ tsp. dry yeast, active
- 1 tbsp. brown sugar
- 2 tsp. salt
- 1 tsp. ground cinnamon
- ¾ cup chopped walnuts
- ¾ cup dried cranberries

Directions:

1. Gather all the ingredients needed for the bread.
2. Power on bread machine that has about 2 pounds of the bread pan.
3. Add all the ingredients except for nuts and cranberries into the bread machine pan in the order mentioned in the ingredients list.
4. Press the "Dough" button, press the start button, let mixture knead for 5 minutes, then add walnuts and cranberries and continue kneading for 5 minutes until

all the ingredients have thoroughly combined and incorporated.

5. Select the "basic/white" cycle, press the up/down arrow to set baking time to 4 hours.

6. Select light or medium color for the crust, and press the start button.

7. Then carefully lift the bread, and transfer it to a wire rack for 1 hour or additional until cooled.

8. Cut bread into slices and then serve.

Nutrition:

Calories: 134

Fat (g): 3

Protein (g): 4

Carbs: 24

31.   Pumpkin Bread with Walnuts

Preparation Time: 10 Minutes

Cooking Time: 1 Hour

Servings: 16

Ingredients:

- 2/3 cup olive oil
- 1 1/3 cups pumpkin puree
- 2 ¾ eggs, at room temperature
- 2 cups all-purpose flour
- ¼ tsp. baking powder
- 1 ¼ tsp. baking soda
- 1/4 tsp. ground ginger
- 2 cups sugar
- 1 tsp. salt
- ¾ tsp. ground cinnamon
- ¾ tsp. ground nutmeg
- chopped walnuts

Directions:

1. Gather all the ingredients needed for the bread.
2. Power on bread machine that has about 2 pounds of the bread pan.
3. Take a large mixing bowl, add eggs to it and then beat in sugar, oil, and pumpkin puree using an electric mixer until smooth and well blended.

4. Beat in salt, all the spices, baking powder, and soda, and then beat in flour, ½-cup at a time, until incorporated.

5. Pour the batter into the bread pan, top with nuts, select the "cake/quick bread" cycle, or press the up/down arrow to set baking time to 1 hour.

6. Choose light or medium color for the crust, and then press the start button.

7. Then carefully get out the bread and hand it to a wire rack for 1 hour or more until cooled.

8. Cut bread into sixteen slices and then serve.

Nutrition:

Calories: 166

Fat (g): 9

Protein (g): 3

Carbs: 19g

Meat Breads
and
Pizza Dough

32.   French Ham Bread

Preparation Time: 30-45 Minutes

Cooking Time: 2 Hours

Servings: 8

Ingredients:

- 3 1/3 cups wheat flour
- 1 cup ham
- ½ cup of milk powder
- 1 ½ tablespoons sugar
- One teaspoon yeast, fresh
- One teaspoon salt
- One teaspoon dried basil
- 1 1/3 cups water
- Two tablespoons olive oil

Directions:

1. Cut ham into cubes of 0.5-1 cm (approximately ¼ inch).

2. Put the bread maker's fixings in the following order: water, olive oil, salt, sugar, flour, milk powder, ham, and yeast.
3. Put all the ingredients rendering to the instructions in your bread maker.
4. Basil put in a dispenser or fill it later, at the signal in the container.
5. Turn on the bread maker.
6. After the end of the baking cycle, leave the bread container
7. in the bread maker to keep warm for 1 hour.
8. Then your delicious bread is ready!

Nutrition:

Calories 287

Total Fat 5.5g

Saturated Fat 1.1g

Cholesterol 11g

Sodium 557mg

Total Carbohydrate 47.2g

Dietary Fiber 1.7g

Total Sugars 6.4g

Protein 11.4g

33. Meat Bread

Preparation Time: 1 Hour and 30 Minutes

Cooking Time: 1 Hour and 30 Minutes

Servings: 8

Ingredients:

- 2 cups boiled chicken
- 1 cup milk
- 3 cups flour
- One tablespoon dry yeast
- One egg
- One teaspoon sugar
- ½ tablespoon salt
- Two tablespoons oil

Directions:

1. Pre-cook the meat. You can use a leg or fillet.
2. Distinct the meat from the bone and cut it into small pieces.
3. Pour all ingredients into the bread maker according to the instructions.
4. Add chicken pieces now.
5. Then set the machine to the setting for Basic or White Bread and push the start button.
6. This bread is perfectly combined with dill and butter.

Nutrition:

Calories 283

Total Fat 6.2g

Saturated Fat 1.4g

Cholesterol 50g

Sodium 484mg

Total Carbohydrate 38.4g

Dietary Fiber 1.6g

Total Sugars 2g

Protein 17.2g

34.   Onion Bacon Bread

Preparation Time: 1 Hour and 30 Minutes

Cooking Time: 1 Hour and 30 Minutes

Servings: 8

Ingredients:

- 1 ½ cups water
- Two tablespoons sugar
- Three teaspoons dry yeast
- 4 ½ cups flour
- One egg
- Two teaspoons salt
- One tablespoon oil
- Three small onions, chopped
- 1 cup bacon

Directions:

1. Cut the bacon.
2. Put all the ingredients into the machine.
3. Set it to the Basic program.
4. Enjoy this tasty bread!

Nutrition:

Calories 391	**Total Fat** 9.7g
Saturated Fat 2.7g	**Cholesterol** 38g
Sodium 960mg	**Total Carbohydrate** 59.9g
Dietary Fiber 2.8g	**Total Sugars** 4.3g
Protein 14.7g	

35.   Fish Bell Pepper Bran Bread

Preparation Time: 1 Hour and 30 Minutes

Cooking Time: 1 Hour and 30 Minutes

Servings: 8

Ingredients:

- 2 ½ cups flour
- ½ cup bran
- 1 1/3 cups water
- 1 ½ teaspoons salt
- 1 ½ teaspoons sugar
- 1 ½ tablespoon mustard oil
- One ¼ teaspoons dry yeast
- Two teaspoons powdered milk
- 1 cup chopped bell pepper
- ¾ cup chopped smoked fish
- One onion

Directions:

1.   Mix flour, bran, water, sugar and yeast in a large bowl.

2. Add salt, mustard oil and milk powder to the mixture. Mix well and stir for five minutes or until smooth.

3. Add chopped bell pepper, fish and onion to the mixture and stir until well combined.

4. Transfer the dough to a greased baking dish and allow it to rise for one hour or slightly longer.

5. Preheat your oven to 350 degrees F after one hour or when the dough is ready.

6. Punch down the dough and bake for 70 minutes; you can reduce the heat to 300 degrees F after 30 minutes. Transfer from the baking dish to a wire rack and allow it to completely cool.

Nutrition:

Calories 208

Total Fat 3.8g

Saturated Fat 0.5g

Cholesterol 8g

Sodium 487mg

Total Carbohydrate 35.9g

Dietary Fiber 4.2g

Total Sugars 2.7g

Protein 7.2g

36.   Sausage Bread

Preparation Time: 2 Hours

Cooking Time: 2 Hours

Servings: 8

Ingredients:

- 1 ½ teaspoons dry yeast
- 3 cups flour
- One teaspoon sugar
- 1 ½ teaspoons salt
- 1 1/3 cups whey
- One tablespoon oil
- 1 cup chopped smoked sausage

Directions:

1. Fold all the ingredients in the order that is recommended specifically for your model.
2. Set the required parameters for baking bread.
3. When ready, remove the delicious hot bread.
4. Wait for it to cool down and enjoy sausage.

Nutrition:

Calories 234   **Total Fat** 5.1g

Saturated Fat 1.2g   **Cholesterol** 9g

Sodium 535mg

Total Carbohydrate 38.7g

Dietary Fiber 1.4g

Total Sugars 2.7g

Protein 7.4g

37. Cheese Sausage Bread

Preparation Time: 2 Hours

Cooking Time: 2 Hours

Servings: 8

Ingredients:

- One teaspoon dry yeast
- 3 ½ cups flour
- One teaspoon salt
- One tablespoon sugar
- 1 ½ tablespoon oil
- Two tablespoons smoked sausage
- Two tablespoons grated cheese
- One tablespoon chopped garlic
- 1 cup of water

Directions:

1. Cut the sausage into small cubes.
2. Grate the cheese on a grater
3. chop the garlic.
4. Add the ingredients to the bread machine, rendering to the instructions.
5. Turn on the baking program, and let it do the work.

Nutrition:

Calories 260

Total Fat 5.6g

Saturated Fat 1.4g

Cholesterol 8g

Sodium 355mg

Total Carbohydrate 43.8g

Dietary Fiber 1.6g

Total Sugars 1.7g

Protein 7.7g

38.   Cheesy Pizza Dough

Preparation Time: 20 Minutes

Cooking Time: 1 Hour and 30 Minutes

Servings: 4

Ingredients:

- 1/2 cup warm beer, or more as needed
- 1 tbsp. Parmesan cheese
- 1 1/2 tsp. pizza dough yeast
- 1 tsp. salt
- 1 tsp. ground black pepper
- 1 tsp. granulated garlic
- 1 tbsp. olive oil
- 1 1/4 cups all-purpose flour

Directions:

1. In a big mixing bowl, mix granulated garlic, pepper, salt, yeast, Parmesan cheese, and beer. Mix until salt dissolves. Allow mixture to stand for 10-20 minutes until yeast creates a creamy layer. Mix in olive oil.

2. Mix flour in yeast mixture until dough becomes smooth. Add small amounts of flour or beer if the dough is too sticky or dry. Let rise for an hour. Punch dough down, then roll out into a pizza crust on a work surface that's floured.

Nutrition:

Calories: 199

Total Carbohydrate: 32.4 g

Cholesterol: 1 mg

Total Fat: 4.2 g

Protein: 5.4 g

Sodium: 604 mg

39. Collards and Bacon Grilled Pizza

Preparation Time: 15 Minutes

Cooking Time: 15 Minutes

Servings: 4

Ingredients:

- 1 lb. whole-wheat pizza dough
- 3 tbsp. garlic-flavored olive oil
- 2 cups thinly sliced cooked collard greens
- 1 cup shredded Cheddar cheese
- ¼ cup crumbled cooked bacon

Directions:

1. Heat grill to medium-high.
2. Roll out dough to an oval that's 12 inches on a surface that's lightly floured. Move to a big baking sheet that's lightly floured. Put Cheddar, collards, oil, and dough on the grill.
3. Grease grill rack. Move crust to grill. Close the lid and cook for 1-2 minutes until lightly brown and puffed. Use tongs to flip over the crust—spread oil on the crust and top with Cheddar and collards. Close lid and cook until cheese melts for another 2-3 minutes or the crust is light brown at the bottom.
4. Put pizza on the baking sheet and top using bacon.

Nutrition:

Calories: 498

Total Carbohydrate: 50 g

Cholesterol: 33 mg

Total Fat: 28 g

Fiber: 6 g

Protein: 19 g

Sodium: 573 mg

Sugar: 3 g

Saturated Fat: 7 g

40. Crazy Cut Pizza Dough

Preparation Time: 10 Minutes

Cooking Time: 45 Minutes

Servings: 8

Ingredients:

- 1 cup all-purpose flour
- 1 tsp. salt
- 1 tsp. dried oregano
- 1/8 tsp. black pepper
- Two eggs, lightly beaten
- 2/3 cup milk

Directions:

1. Heat oven, then grease a baking sheet or rimmed pizza pan lightly.

2. Mix the black pepper, oregano, salt, and flour in a big bowl. Stir in milk and eggs thoroughly. Put butter in the pan and tilt it until it is evenly coated. Put at all toppings you want on top of the batter.

3. Next is baking it in the oven until the crust is set for 20-25 minutes.

4. Take the crust out of the oven. Drizzle pizza sauce on and top with cheese. Bake for around 10 minutes until the cheese melts.

Nutrition:

Calories: 86

Total Carbohydrate: 13.1 g

Cholesterol: 48 mg

Total Fat: 1.8 g

Protein: 3.9 g

Sodium: 317 mg

41. Deep Dish Pizza Dough

Preparation Time: 15 Minutes

Cooking Time: 2 Hours and 15 Minutes

Servings: 8

Ingredients:

- 1 (.25 oz.) package active dry yeast
- 1/3 cup white sugar
- 2/3 cup water
- 2 cups all-purpose flour
- 1 cup bread flour
- 1/4 cup corn oil
- 2 tsp. salt
- 6 tbsp. vegetable oil
- 1/2 cup all-purpose flour

Directions:

1. Dissolve sugar and yeast in a bowl with water. Let the mixture stand for 5 minutes. Wait until the yeast starts to form creamy foam and softens.

2. In a bowl, mix bread flour, salt, corn oil, and 2 cups of all-purpose flour. Add the yeast mixture. Knead the mixture in a work surface using 1/2 of the all-purpose flour until well-incorporated. Place the dough in a warm area, then wait for it rises for 2 hours until its size doubles.

Nutrition:

Calories: 328

Total Carbohydrate: 38.5 g

Cholesterol: 0 mg

Total Fat: 17.5 g

Protein: 4.4 g

Sodium: 583 mg

42.   Double Crust Stuffed Pizza

Preparation Time: 30 Minutes

Cooking Time: 2 Hours and 45 Minutes

Servings: 8

Ingredients:

- 1 1/2 tsp. white sugar
- 1 cup of warm water
- 1 1/2 tsp. active dry yeast
- 1 tbsp. olive oil
- 1/2 tsp. salt
- 2 cups all-purpose flour
- 1 (8 oz.) can crushed tomatoes
- 1 tbsp. packed brown sugar
- 1/2 tsp. garlic powder
- 1 tsp. olive oil
- 1/2 tsp. salt
- 3 cups shredded mozzarella cheese, divided
- 1/2 lb. bulk Italian sausage
- 1 (4 oz.) package sliced pepperoni
- 1 (8 oz.) package sliced fresh mushrooms
- 1/2 green bell pepper, chopped
- 1/2 red bell pepper, chopped

Directions:

1. Mix warm water and white sugar. Sprinkle with yeast and let the mixture stand for 5 minutes until the yeast

starts to form creamy foam and softens. Stir in 1 tbsp. of olive oil.

2. Mix flour with 1/2 tsp. of salt. Put half of the flour mix into the yeast mixture and mix until no dry spots are visible. Whisk in remaining flour, a half cup at a time, mixing well every after addition. Place the dough on a lightly floured surface once it has pulled together. Knead the dough for 8 minutes until elastic and smooth. You can use the dough hook in a stand mixer to mix the dough.

3. Move the dough into a lightly oiled large bowl and flip to coat the dough with oil. Use a light cloth to cover the dough. Let it rise in a warm place for 1 hour until the volume doubles.

4. In a small saucepan, mix 1 tsp. of olive oil, brown sugar, crushed tomatoes, garlic powder, and salt. Cover the saucepan, then cook over low heat for 30 minutes until the tomatoes begin to break down.

5. Set the oven to 450°F (230°C) for preheating. Compress the dough and place it on a lightly floured surface. Divide the dough into two equal portions, then roll one part into a 12-inches thin circle. Roll the other part into a 9-inches thicker circle.

6. Press the 12-inches dough round into an ungreased 9-inches springform pan. Top the dough with a cup of cheese. Form sausage into a 9-inches patty and place it

on top of the cheese. Arrange pepperoni, green pepper, mushrooms, red pepper, and remaining cheese on top of the sausage patty. Then place the 9-inches dough round on top, pinching its edges to seal. Make vent holes on top of the crust by cutting several 1/2-inch on top. Pour the sauce evenly on top of the crust, leaving an only 1/2-inch border at the edges.

7. Bake the pizza inside the preheated oven for 40-45 minutes. Wait until the cheese is melted, the sausage is cooked through, and the crust is fixed. Let the pizza rest for 15 minutes. Before serving, cut the pizza into wedges.

Nutrition:

Calories: 410

Total Carbohydrate: 32.5 g

Cholesterol: 53 mg

Total Fat: 21.1 g

Protein: 22.2 g

Sodium: 1063 mg

43. Chicken Bread

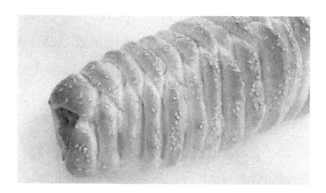

Chicken bread is not only delicious, but it's a great source of protein and excellent for children's health. Why not give it a try for yourself?

Preparation time: 15 minutes

Cooking time: 3 hours & 30 minutes

Servings: 10

Ingredients:

- 2 cups boiled chicken, chopped
- 1 cup lukewarm whole milk
- 3 cups of wheat bread machine flour, sifted
- 1 tbsp. bread machine yeast
- 1 whole egg
- 1 tsp. sugar
- ½ tbsp. sea salt
- 2 tbsp. extra-virgin olive oil
-

Directions:

1. Pre-cook the chicken. You'll use a leg or fillet. Separate the chicken from the bone and cut it into small pieces.

2. Place all the dry and liquid ingredients, except the chicken, in the pan, and follow the bread machine's instructions.

3. Set the baking program to Basic and, therefore, the crust type to Medium. Add the chicken after the beep or place them in the dispenser of the bread machine.

4. If your dough is too dense or too wet, adjust the recipe's flour and liquid quantity. When the program has ended, take the pan out of the bread machine and cool for 5 minutes.

5. Shake the loaf out of the pan. If necessary, use a spatula. Wrap the bread with a kitchen towel and set it aside for an hour. Otherwise, you'll calm on a wire rack.

Nutrition:

Calories 283

Fat 6.2g

Carbohydrate 38.4g

Protein 17.2g

44.   Beef and Parmesan Bread

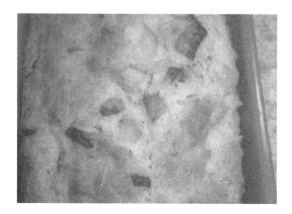

Bread with Beef and Parmesan is an innovation in bread making. It is an innovative way to have some great tasting bread whenever you please.

Preparation time: 1 hour

Cooking time: 1 hour

Servings: 6

Ingredients:

- 10 oz beef
- 1 cup of Parmesan cheese, grated
- 1 cup of wheat flour
- 1 cup of rye flour
- 2 onions
- 3 teaspoons dry yeast
- 5 tablespoons olive oil
- Sea salt to taste

- black pepper to taste
- red pepper to taste
- 1 teaspoon basilica

Directions:

1. Pour the warm water into the wheat flour and rye flour and leave overnight. Sprinkle the yeast with the sugar and set aside for 10 minutes. Minced the onions, then cut the beef into small cubes.

2. In a skillet or wok, fry the beef chunks on low heat for around 20 minutes until soft and then mix in the onions and fry until transparent and caramelized.

3. Combine the yeast with the warm water, mixing until smooth consistency, and then combine the yeast with the flour, salt, and basilica, but don't forget to mix and knead well.

4. Add in the fried onions with the beef chunks, Parmesan cheese, black and red pepper, and mix well.

5. Pour some oil into a bread machine and place the dough into the bread maker. Cover the dough with the towel and leave for 1 hour.

6. Close the lid and turn the bread machine on the basic/white bread program.

7. Bake the meat bread until the medium crust, and after the bread is ready, take it out and leave for 1 hour covered with the towel, and slice the bread.

Nutrition:

Calories: 110

Carbs: 14g

Fat: 6g

Protein: 2g

45. Bacon and Walnuts Rye Bread

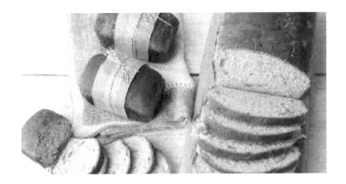

Bacon and Walnuts Rye Bread is a perfect recipe for the bread machine. This delicious combination of bacon and nuts. It is both a good dinner bread and an excellent bread for sandwiches.

Preparation time: overnight & 1 hour

Cooking time: 60 minutes

Servings: 4

Ingredients:

- 7 oz bacon
- 1 cup of walnuts
- 2 big onions
- 15 oz rye flour
- 5 oz wheat flour
- 3 tsp. dry yeast
- 3 tbsp. olive oil
- 1 tbsp. sugar

- Sea salt

Directions:

1. Preheat the oven to 250-270F and roast the walnuts in the oven for 10 minutes until lightly browned and crispy and then set aside to cool completely. Then grind the walnuts using a food processor or blender.

2. Combine the wheat flour and rye flour and pour the warm water to leave overnight. Chop the onions and cut the bacon into cubes.

3. Fry the onions until transparent and caramelized, and then add in the bacon and fry on low heat for around 20 minutes until soft or on medium heat for 15 minutes.

4. Combine the yeast with the warm water, mixing until smooth consistency and then combine the yeast with the rye and wheat flour, walnuts, salt, and sugar, and then mix and knead well.

5. Add in the fried onions with the bacon and mix well. Pour some oil into a bread machine and place the dough into the bread maker. Wrap the dough with the towel and leave for 1 hour.

6. Set to basic/white bread program. Bake the bread until the medium crust, and after the bread is ready, take it out and leave for 1 hour covered with the towel, then slice the bread.

Nutrition:

Calories: 140

Carbs: 28g

Fat: 3g

Protein: 5g

46. Turkey Breast Bread

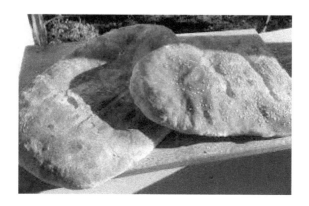

This bread is best when made with leftover turkey breast, but you can use chicken or beef in place of the turkey if your family has a family tradition that doesn't include turkey.

Preparation time: 60 minutes

Cooking time: 60 minutes

Servings: 6

Ingredients:

- 1 smoked turkey breast
- 1 cup of Pecorino cheese, grated
- 2 cups of wheat flour
- 1 cup of rye flour
- 1 cup of raisins
- 10 oz bran
- 4 chopped cloves of garlic
- 2 onions

- 3 teaspoons dry yeast
- 1 cup of warm water
- 2 tablespoons powdered milk
- 2 tablespoons sugar
- 3 tablespoons olive oil
- sea salt
- black pepper

Directions:

1. Chop the onions and fry until transparent and caramelized. Cut the turkey breast into small pieces and combine them with the raisins. Combine all the ingredients and mix until smooth consistency.

2. Pour some oil into a bread machine and place the dough into the bread maker. Wrap the dough using a towel and leave for 1 hour.

3. Set to basic/white bread program. Bake until the medium crust, and after the turkey bread is ready, take it out and leave for few hours on a grate and only then slice.

Nutrition:

Calories: 250

Carbs: 0g

Fat: 12g

Protein: 5g

47. Bread with Chicken, Apricots, and Raisins

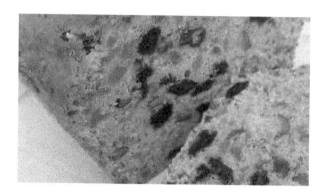

This bread is perfect for those who like eastern touches among their western recipes. Indeed, a combination of tasty favorites!

Preparation time: 60 minutes

Cooking time: 1 hour & 10 minutes

Servings: 6

Ingredients:

- 10 oz chicken chunks
- 1 cup of apricots
- 1 cup of raisins
- 15 oz wheat flour
- 15 oz rye flour
- 4 chopped cloves of garlic
- 2 onions
- 3 teaspoons dry yeast
- 1 cup of warm milk

- 2 tablespoons sugar
- 3 tablespoons olive oil
- Sea salt
- ground black pepper

Directions:

1. Soak the apricots and raisins in the warm water for 10 minutes, and then cube the apricots. Chop the onions and fry until transparent and caramelized.
2. In a skillet or a wok, fry the chicken chunks for around 10 minutes. Combine all the ingredients and mix well.
3. Pour some oil into a bread machine and place the dough into the bread maker. Wrap the dough with the towel and leave for 1 hour. Set to basic/white bread program.
4. Bake until the medium crust, and after the bread is ready, take it out and leave for few hours on a grate and only then slice.

Nutrition:

Calories: 130

Carbs: 32g

Fat: 3g

Protein: 2g

48.   Bread with Beef and Hazelnuts

This bread is so easy to make. You do not need to wait for raising, knead, or proofing. It is very healthy bread. This bread is very popular in the north of Italy in a region called Lombardia.

Preparation time: 60 minutes

Cooking time: 60 minutes

Servings: 6

Ingredients:

- 5 oz beef
- 1 cup of hazelnuts
- 15 oz wheat flour
- 5 oz rye flour
- 1 onion
- 3 teaspoons dry yeast
- 5 tablespoons olive oil
- 1 tablespoon sugar
- Sea salt
- ground black pepper

Directions:

1. Preheat the oven to 250-270 Fahrenheit and roast the hazelnuts in the oven for 10 minutes until lightly browned and crispy and then set aside to cool completely. Then grind the hazelnuts using a food processor or blender.

2. Pour the warm water into the 15 oz of the wheat flour and rye flour and leave overnight. Minced the onions and cut the beef into cubes.

3. Fry the onions until transparent and golden brown and then mix in the bacon and fry on low heat for 20 minutes until soft.

4. Combine the yeast with the warm water, mixing until smooth consistency, and then combine the yeast with the flour, salt and sugar, but don't forget to mix and knead well.

5. Add in the fried onions with the beef, hazelnuts, and black pepper and mix well. Pour some oil into a bread machine, place the dough into the bread maker, wrap the dough with the towel, and leave for 1 hour.

6. Set to basic/white bread program. Bake the bread until the medium crust, and after the bread is ready, take it out and leave for 1 hour covered with the towel, then can slice the bread.

Nutrition:

Calories: 290

Carbs: 42g

Fat: 11g

Protein: 5g

49. Bread with Ham and Sausages

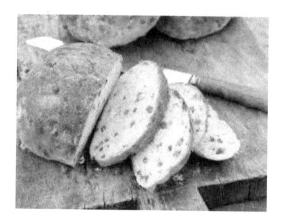

This bread is for all of you who like the taste of meat in your house. It comes out like a sticky bun or cake. It works well toasted. Guaranteed your family will love it.

Preparation time: 60 minutes

Cooking time: 60 minutes

Servings: 8

Ingredients:

- 8 oz ham
- 4 sausages, cubed
- 5 oz Herbes de Provence
- 10 oz wheat flour
- 10 oz rye flour
- 3 teaspoons dry yeast
- 5 oz warm water
- 1 cup of unsalted butter

- ½ half cup of olive oil
- Sea salt
- ground black pepper to taste

Directions:

1. Cut the ham into cubes. Fry the ham for 10-15 minutes on low heat until golden brown, and then mix in the cubed sausages.
2. Combine the unsalted butter with the Herbes de Provence, salt, pepper, and sifted flour, mixing until smooth consistency. Combine the flour mixture with the yeast and mix well.
3. Pour the warm water and the olive oil into the mixture and mix until the dough has a smooth consistency and homogenous mass. Stir in the fried ham and sausages and mix well.
4. Pour some oil into the bread machine and place the dough into the bread maker. Cover the dough with the towel and leave for 1 hour.
5. Set to basic/white bread program. Bake until the medium crust, and after the bread is ready, take it out and leave for few hours on a grate and only then slice.

Nutrition:

Calories: 124

Carbs: 18g

Fat: 1g

Protein: 8g

50. Bread with Sausages and Celery

This bread is perfect for breakfast on a cold winter morning. It has just the right number of calories, and it's loaded with vital vitamins and minerals.

Preparation time: 60 minutes

Cooking time: 60 minutes

Servings: 8

Ingredients:

- 10 sausages
- 1 big celery, cubed
- 10 oz wheat flour
- 10 oz rye flour
- 3 teaspoon dry yeast
- 5 oz warm water
- 1 cup of unsalted butter
- 5 tablespoons olive oil
- Sea salt
- ground black pepper

Directions:

1. Cut the sausages into rings. Fry the sausages for 10-15 minutes on low heat until golden brown and mix in the celery cubes to stew for around 20 minutes on low heat.

2. Combine the unsalted butter with the salt, pepper, and sifted flour, mixing until smooth consistency and

homogenous mass. Combine the flour mixture with the yeast and mix well.

3. Pour the warm water and the olive oil into the mixture and mix until the dough has a smooth consistency. Add the fried sausages with the celery and mix well.

4. Pour some oil into a bread machine and place the dough into the bread maker. Cover the dough with the towel and leave for 1 hour.

5. Set to basic/white bread program. Bake until the medium crust, and after the bread is ready, take it out and leave for few hours on a grate and only then slice.

Nutrition:

Calories: 254

Carbs: 25g

Fat: 16g

Protein: 4g

9 781803 110486